The Silver Yogi:
An Introduction to Yoga for Seniors
Linda Standrige

The Silver Yogi

Linda Standridge

Published by Linda Standridge, 2023.

While every precaution has been taken in the preparation of this book, the publisher assumes no responsibility for errors or omissions, or for damages resulting from the use of the information contained herein.

THE SILVER YOGI

First edition. December 2, 2023.

ISBN: 979-8223701545

Written by Linda Standridge.

Table of Contents

Chapter One:

Understanding the Benefits of Yoga for Seniors

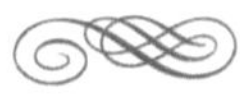

AS WE AGE, IT IS CRUCIAL to prioritize our physical and mental well-being. Yoga has emerged as a powerful tool for promoting holistic wellness among seniors. In this chapter, we will explore the numerous benefits that yoga can offer adults over 60, focusing on the specific niche of yoga for seniors.

Improved flexibility and balance: Aging often leads to decreased flexibility and balance, making seniors susceptible to falls and injuries. Yoga helps seniors regain and maintain their flexibility, enhancing their range of motion. Regular practice also strengthens the muscles and improves balance, reducing the risk of falls and promoting overall stability.

Stress relief and mental well-being: Yoga is renowned for its stress-relieving properties. Yoga provides a safe space for seniors facing various life transitions and challenges to unwind and find inner peace. Combining physical postures, breathing exercises, and meditation promotes relaxation, reduces anxiety, and enhances mental well-being.

Enhanced joint health: Arthritis and joint pain are common issues among seniors. Yoga offers gentle movements to lubricate joints, promoting health and reducing discomfort. The low-impact nature of yoga makes it an ideal exercise option for seniors with joint issues, allowing them to improve their mobility without putting excessive strain on their bodies.

Increased strength and stamina: Regular yoga practice helps seniors build strength in their muscles, allowing them to perform daily activities with ease. The gentle stretching and holding poses contribute to muscle toning and overall endurance. As seniors become stronger, they often experience a renewed sense of vitality and energy.

Social connection: Practicing in yoga classes for seniors fosters a sense of community and social connection. Seniors can connect with like-minded individuals, sharing their experiences and forming meaningful friendships. The supportive environment of a yoga class encourages seniors to stay motivated and committed to their wellness journey.

Better Sleep: Sleep disturbances are common among older adults. Yoga's emphasis on relaxation and mindfulness can greatly improve sleep quality. Incorporating a bedtime yoga routine can help seniors unwind, release tension, and promote a restful night's sleep.

In summary, yoga offers a multitude of benefits for seniors, addressing their unique physical, mental, and emotional needs. By embracing yoga as a holistic wellness practice, seniors can enjoy improved flexibility, balance, joint health, strength, and stamina. Additionally, yoga promotes stress relief, mental well-being, social connections, and better sleep. It is never too late to begin a yoga journey and reap its incredible rewards for seniors seeking a healthier and more fulfilling life.

Overcoming Age-Related Challenges in Yoga Practice

As we age, our bodies go through various changes that can present challenges when it comes to practicing yoga. However, it is essential to understand that yoga is for everyone, regardless of age or physical condition. With a few modifications and a mindful approach, adults over 60 can continue to reap the countless benefits of yoga practice.

One common challenge that seniors may face is reduced flexibility and joint stiffness. This can make performing certain poses or moving fluidly on the mat difficult. The key here is to listen to your body and honor its limitations. Focus on gentle stretching exercises that target specific areas of stiffness, such as hips or shoulders. Over time, with regular practice, you will notice an improvement in your flexibility and range of motion.

Another challenge seniors may encounter is balance issues. Aging can affect our sense of balance, making it more challenging to maintain a steady footing during yoga poses. It is crucial to prioritize safety in your practice by utilizing props such as blocks of a sturdy chair for support. Incorporating balance exercises, like tree poses or standing on one leg, can also help improve stability and coordination over time.

Additionally, older adults may experience a decrease in strength and muscle mass. This can make it challenging to hold certain poses or maintain proper alignment. To overcome this challenge, focus on building strength gradually through gentle strength-training exercises. Incorporate props like resistance bands or light weights and gradually increase as you feel comfortable.

Lastly, it is essential to be mindful of any existing health conditions or injuries that may require modifications in your yoga practice. Always consult with your healthcare provider before starting a new exercise regimen, including yoga. They can provide guidance on specific modifications or alternate poses that will be safe and beneficial for your unique circumstances.

Remember, yoga is a holistic practice that goes beyond the physical aspect. It encompasses the mind, body, and spirit. By embracing a mindful approach, seniors can continue to enjoy the numerous benefits of yoga, including improved flexibility, balance, strength, and overall well-being. With patience, perseverance, and a willingness to adapt, age-related challenges can be overcome, allowing you to embark on a fulfilling yoga journey well into your golden years.

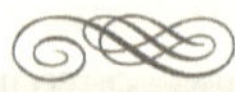

The Importance of Holistic Wellness in the Senior Years

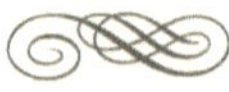

AS WE AGE, IT BECOMES increasingly important to prioritize our overall well-being. Seniors often face unique challenges, both physical and emotional, that can impact their quality of life. This is where the concept of holistic wellness comes into play. We will delve into the significance of holistic wellness in the senior years and how yoga can be a powerful tool for achieving it.

Holistic wellness refers to the integration of physical, mental, and emotional aspects of health. It recognizes that all these elements are interconnected and that neglecting one can affect the others. For seniors, maintaining a balanced and holistic approach to wellness is crucial for leading a fulfilling and healthy life.

Physical well-being is at the forefront of holistic wellness. Engaging in regular exercise, such as yoga, can help seniors improve flexibility, strength, and balance. Yoga postures tailored specifically for seniors can alleviate joint pain, increase mobility, and enhance overall physical functioning. By incorporating gentle movements and breathing exercises, yoga promotes circulation, boosts immunity, and reduces the risk of age-related ailments.

Mental and emotional well-being are equally vital in the senior years. Yoga offers a unique opportunity to cultivate mindfulness and reduce stress. Through various breathing techniques and meditation, seniors can develop a sense of inner calm, reduce anxiety, and enhance their ability to cope with life's challenges. Additionally, yoga can improve cognitive function, memory, and overall mental clarity.

The social aspect of holistic wellness should not be overlooked either. Participating in group classes allows seniors to connect with like-minded individuals and build a supportive community. This sense of belonging fosters emotional well-being and combats feelings of loneliness and isolation, which are common among older adults.

In conclusion, holistic wellness is of utmost importance in the senior years. By embracing a holistic approach to well-being through yoga, seniors can experience a multitude of benefits. From physical improvements to mental clarity and emotional balance, yoga offers a comprehensive solution for seniors looking to enhance their quality of life. So, let us embark on this journey of holistic wellness, where the silver years can truly become a time of growth, vitality, and serenity.

Chapter Two:

Getting Started with Yoga for Seniors

Choosing the Right Yoga Style for Seniors

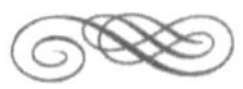

AS WE AGE, IT IS ESSENTIAL to prioritize our overall well-being, and practicing yoga is an excellent way to achieve holistic wellness. However, with the numerous yoga styles available, it can be overwhelming for seniors to determine which one is most suitable for their unique needs. We will explore different yoga styles and help you choose the right one to embark on your yoga journey.

Hatha Yoga:

Hatha Yoga is a gentle and slow-paced style that focuses on breathing techniques and stretching exercises. It is an ideal choice for beginners or seniors with limited mobility. Hatha yoga promotes relaxation, improves flexibility, and enhances balance and posture.

Chair Yoga:

If you have difficulty getting on the floor or have physical limitations, chair yoga is a perfect solution. This style adapts traditional yoga poses to be performed while seated or using a chair for support. Chair yoga improves strength, flexibility, and circulation, making it accessible for individuals with mobility challenges.

Restorative Yoga:

Restorative yoga is a deeply relaxing and gentle practice that utilizes props such as blankets and bolsters to support the body in various poses. It helps seniors release tension, reduce stress, and improve overall well-being. Restorative yoga is particularly beneficial for those recovering from injuries or experiencing chronic pain.

Gentle Yoga:

Gentle yoga, as the name suggests, involves slow and mindful movements, making it an excellent choice for seniors with limited flexibility or joint issues. This style focuses on promoting relaxation and relieving stiffness, making it suitable for individuals with arthritis or age-related conditions.

Yin Yoga:

Yin Yoga involves holding poses for an extended period, typically targeting the connective tissues and joints. This style improves flexibility, increases circulation, and promotes a calm mind. Yin yoga is beneficial for seniors looking to enhance their range of motion and find meditative practice.

When choosing the right yoga style for seniors, it is crucial to listen to your body and consult with a qualified yoga instructor. They can guide you in finding the style that suits your abilities and address any specific concerns or limitations you may have. Remember, the journey of yoga is unique for everyone, and finding the right style will help you embrace the transformative power of yoga in your golden years.

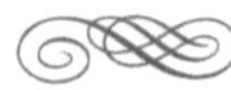

Setting Realistic Goals for Your Yoga Practice

AS ADULTS OVER 60, engaging in a regular yoga practice can greatly enhance our physical and mental well-being. However, it is important to set realistic goals that align with our age, abilities, and health conditions. By doing so, we can experience the numerous benefits of yoga while avoiding unnecessary strain or injury.

One of the key aspects of setting realistic goals for our yoga practice is understanding our personal limitations. As seniors, our bodies may not be as flexible or strong as they once were, and that's okay. Instead of comparing ourselves to others or pushing ourselves beyond our limits, it is crucial to focus on our own journey and progress.

When setting goals, it is essential to take into account any pre-existing health conditions or injuries. Consult with a healthcare professional or a qualified yoga instructor to identify any modifications of specific poses that can be beneficial for your unique circumstances. By doing so, we can tailor our practice and avoid exacerbating any existing issues.

Another important factor in setting realistic goals is acknowledging that progress may be slower compared to when we were younger. Aging affects our bodies differently, and it is essential to be patient and listen to our bodies. Embrace the process and focus on the present moment, rather than solely striving for end results. Celebrate small victories and improvements, as they contribute to our overall well-being.

It is also beneficial to set goals that encompass the mind-body connection. Yoga is not just about physical fitness but also about mental and emotional well-being. Consider incorporating goals related to stress reduction, mindfulness, or cultivating a sense of inner peace. By nurturing the mind-body connection, we can experience a holistic approach to wellness and enhance our overall quality of life.

Lastly, remember that a yoga practice is a personal journey, and each individual's goals may vary. Do not feel pressured to achieve certain poses or levels of flexibility. Instead, focus on how your practice makes you feel and the positive impact it has on your overall well-being.

In conclusion, as adults over 60, setting realistic goals for our yoga practice is crucial. By understanding our limitations, considering our health conditions, being patient with our progress, embracing the mind-body connection, and focusing on our personal journey, we can experience the full benefits of yoga while taking care of our bodies and minds. Let your yoga practice be a source of joy, vitality, and holistic wellness as you navigate the golden years of life.

Creating a Safe and Supportive Environment for Yoga

As adults over 60, it is important for us to prioritize our physical and mental well-being. Yoga can be a wonderful practice to cultivate holistic wellness, but it is crucial to create a safe and supportive environment to fully reap the benefits. We will explore some essential considerations when practicing yoga as seniors.

Firstly, it is essential to find a qualified instructor who specializes in yoga for seniors. Look for someone who understands the unique needs and limitations that come with aging bodies. A knowledgeable instructor will guide you through modifications and adjustments tailored to your specific abilities, ensuring a safe and effective practice.

When setting up your practice space, make sure it is free from potential hazards. Clear away any clutter or tripping hazards, and ensure that the flooring is non-slip. Utilize props such as yoga blocks, straps, and bolsters to support and enhance your practice. These props provide stability and help maintain proper alignment while reducing the risk of injury.

It is also important to listen to your body and honor its limits. As we age, our bodies may not be as flexible or strong as they once were. Be patient and allow yourself to progress at your own pace. Avoid comparing yourself to others and focus on your own progress and growth. Remember that yoga is a personal journey, and each individual's practice is unique.

Maintaining an open line of communication with your instructor is vital. Inform them about any pre-existing medical conditions, injuries, or concerns you may have. This allows them to tailor the practice to your specific needs and provide appropriate modifications. Additionally, do not hesitate to ask questions or seek clarification during the class. Your instructor is there to guide and support you.

Lastly, creating a supportive community can greatly enhance your yoga experience. Engage in conversations with fellow practitioners, share your challenges and successes, and offer support to one another. Participating in group classes or joining yoga communities can provide a sense of camaraderie and motivation.

By creating a safe and supportive environment for yoga, we can fully embrace the benefits of this practice. Remember, yoga is not about achieving perfection or pushing our bodies beyond limits; it is about nurturing ourselves and finding balance in body, mind, and spirit.

Chapter Three:

Essential Yoga Poses for Seniors

Gentle Warm-up Poses for Increased Flexibility

As we age, maintaining flexibility becomes increasingly important for our overall well-being. Yoga offers a gentle and effective way for seniors to improve flexibility, enhance mobility, and promote a sense of balance and harmony in their lives. We will explore some gentle warm-up poses specifically designed for adults over 60, to help you ease into your yoga practice and prepare your body for deeper stretches and movements.

Neck Rolls:

Begin by sitting comfortably with a straight spine. Slowly drop your chin to your chest, and then roll your head gently from one side to the other, making a smooth circular motion. This gentle warm-up pose helps release tension in the neck and shoulders and prepares you for the practice ahead.

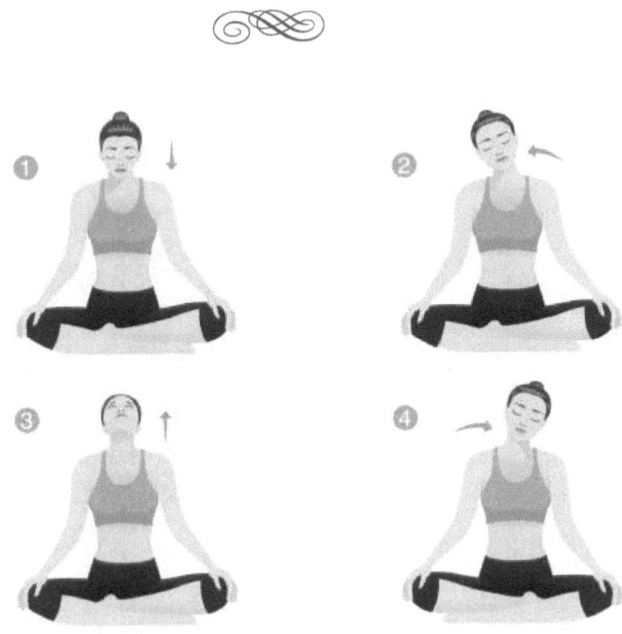

SHOULDER ROLLS:

Stand tall with your feet hip-width apart. Inhale deeply, then exhale as you roll your shoulder backward and downward in a circular motion. This movement helps release tension in the upper body and promotes flexibility in the shoulders and chest.

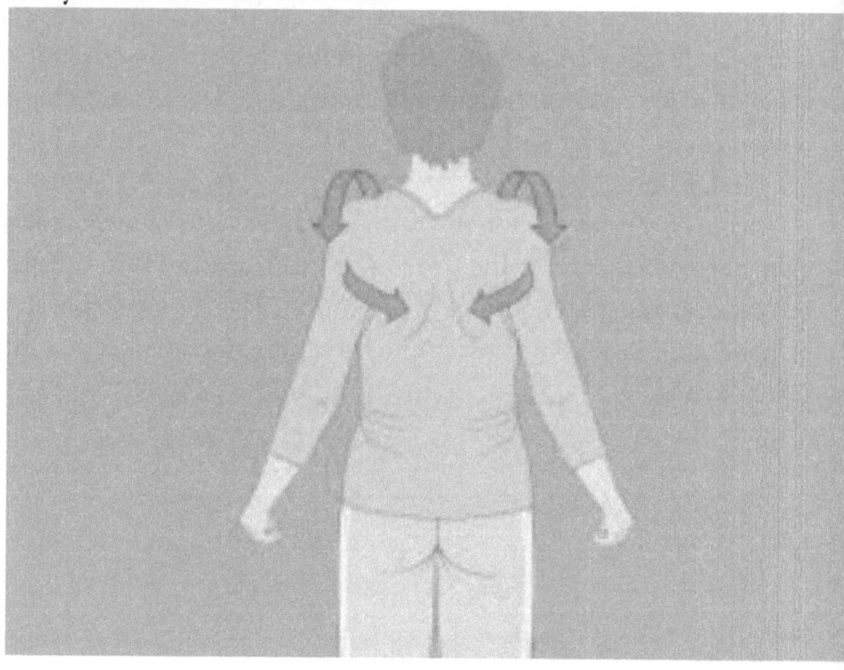

Cat-Cow Pose:

Come onto all fours with your hands directly under your shoulders and knees under your hips. Inhale deeply as you arch your back, lifting your chest and tailbone upwards (Cow Pose). Exhale as you round your spine, tucking your tailbone and dropping your head (Cat Pose). Repeat this gentle flow several, synchronizing your breath with the movement. This pose improves spinal flexibility and gently stretches the back.

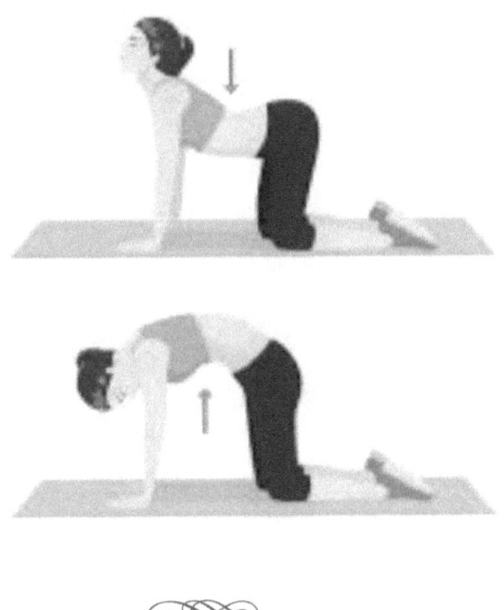

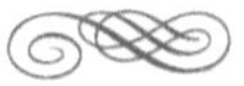

FORWARD FOLD:

Sit on a chair or a bolster with your feet firmly planted on the ground. Inhale deeply, then exhale as you slowly fold forward from your hips, allowing your head to hang gently. Rest your hands on your thighs or reach for your shins, depending on your comfort level. This pose helps stretch the hamstrings and lower back while increasing flexibility in the spine.

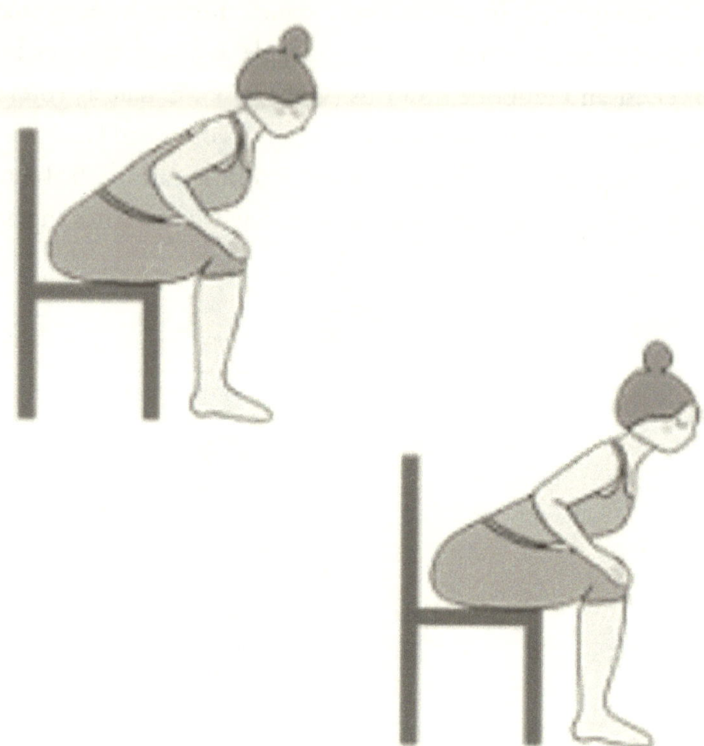

REMEMBER TO MOVE SLOWLY and mindfully throughout your practice, honoring any limitations your body may have. Stay connected to your breath and listen to your body's signals. Over time, with consistent practice, these gentle warm-up poses will help you increase your flexibility, improve your range of motion, and enhance your overall well-being.

Always consult with a qualified yoga instructor or healthcare professional before starting any new exercise program, especially if you have any pre-existing medical conditions or physical limitations.

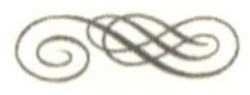

Balancing Poses for Improved Stability and Coordination

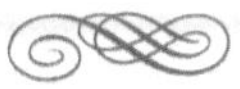

AS WE AGE, MAINTAINING stability and coordination becomes increasingly important for our overall well-being. One of the most effective ways to achieve this is through the practice of yoga. We will explore a range of balancing poses specifically tailored to seniors over 60, helping you enhance your stability and coordination while enjoying the numerous benefits of yoga.

Tree Pose (Vrikshasana):

This pose is perfect for improving balance and strengthening the legs. Stand tall, ground one foot firmly into the floor, and place the sole of the opposite foot against the inner thigh or calf. Find your balance, elongate your spine, and bring your hands to prayer position at your heart. You may use a chair to balance your knee on if needed. Breathe deeply and hold for 30 seconds on each side.

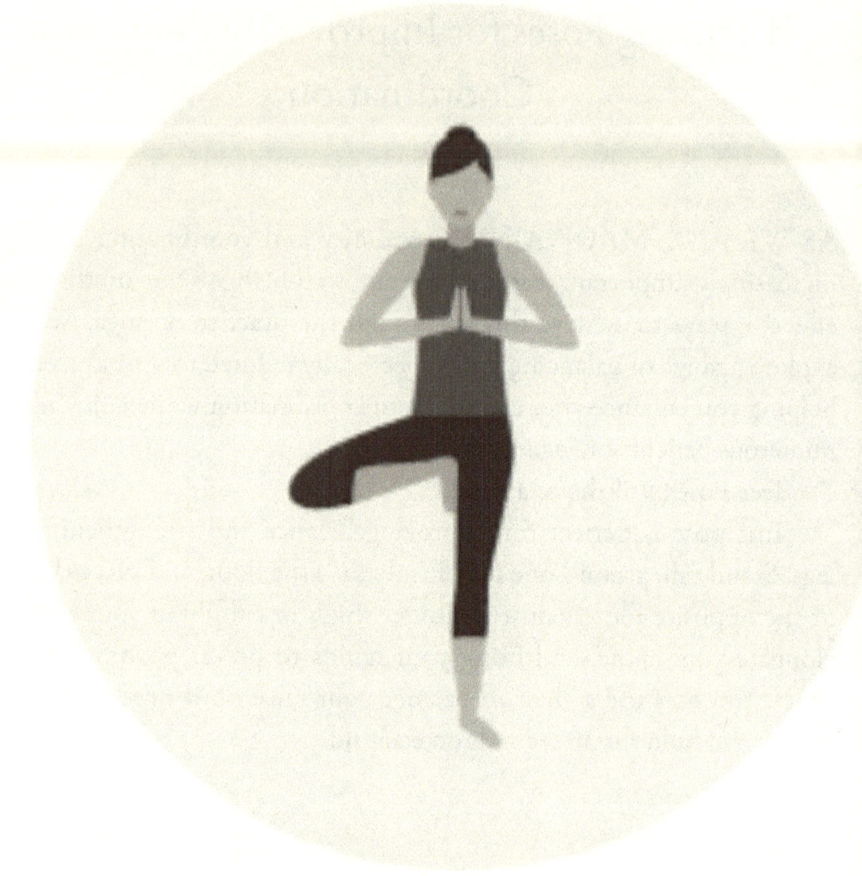

Eagle Pose (Garudasana):

Eagle Pose challenges your balance while stretching your shoulders and hips. Begin by standing tall and crossing your right thigh over your left thigh. Wrap your right foot around your left calf if possible. Bring your arms out in front of you, crossing your right arm over your left, and bend your elbows to bring your palms together. Hold for 30 seconds on each side. You can sit in a chair if needed and follow the steps above.

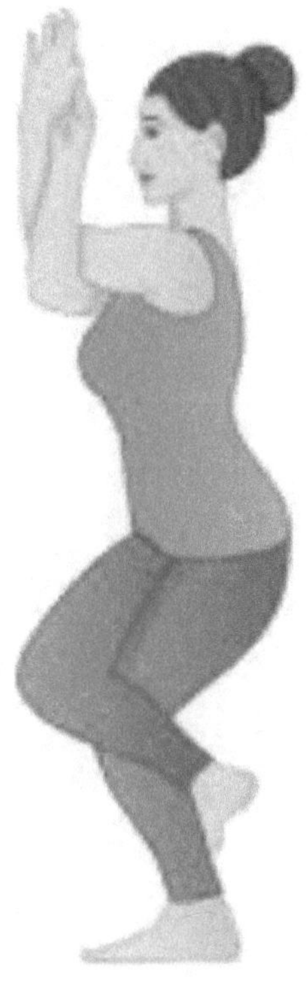

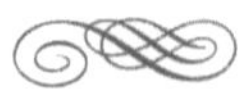

WARRIOR III (VIRABHADRASANA III):

This pose strengthens your legs, and core, and improves overall stability. Start by standing tall and shifting your weight onto your right foot. Extend your left leg behind you, keeping it parallel to the floor

Reach your arms forward or place them on your hips for support. Engage your core and hold for 30 seconds before switching sides. If needed you may hold on to a chair and place your heel against the wall for balance.

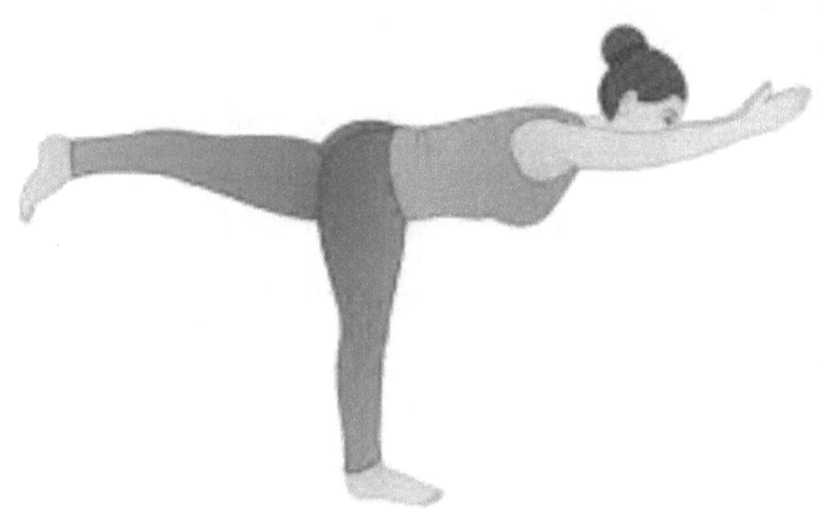

Half Moon Pose (Ardha Chandrasana):

This pose improves balance, and coordination, and strengthens the legs. Begin by standing tall and extending your right leg behind you. Place your right hand on a block or the floor and if needed place your heel against a wall, and simultaneously raise your left arm toward the ceiling. Open your chest and gaze up toward your left hand. Hold for 30 seconds before switching sides.

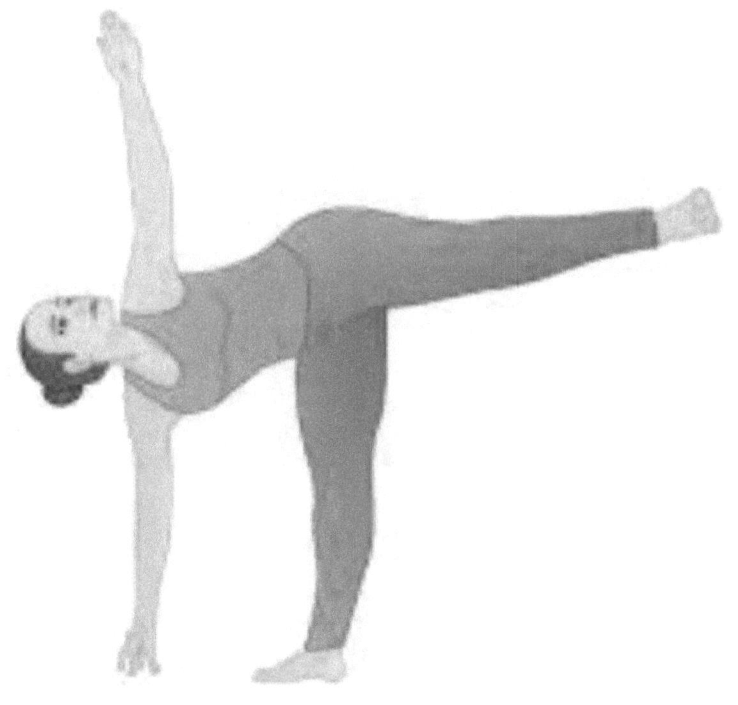

Standing Forward Bend (Uttanasana):

This pose improves balance and flexibility, while also calming the mind. Stand with your feet hip-distance apart, exhale, and fold forward from your hips, allowing your upper body to hang toward the ground. Place your hands on the floor or grab opposite elbows and gently sway side to side. Hold for 30 seconds.

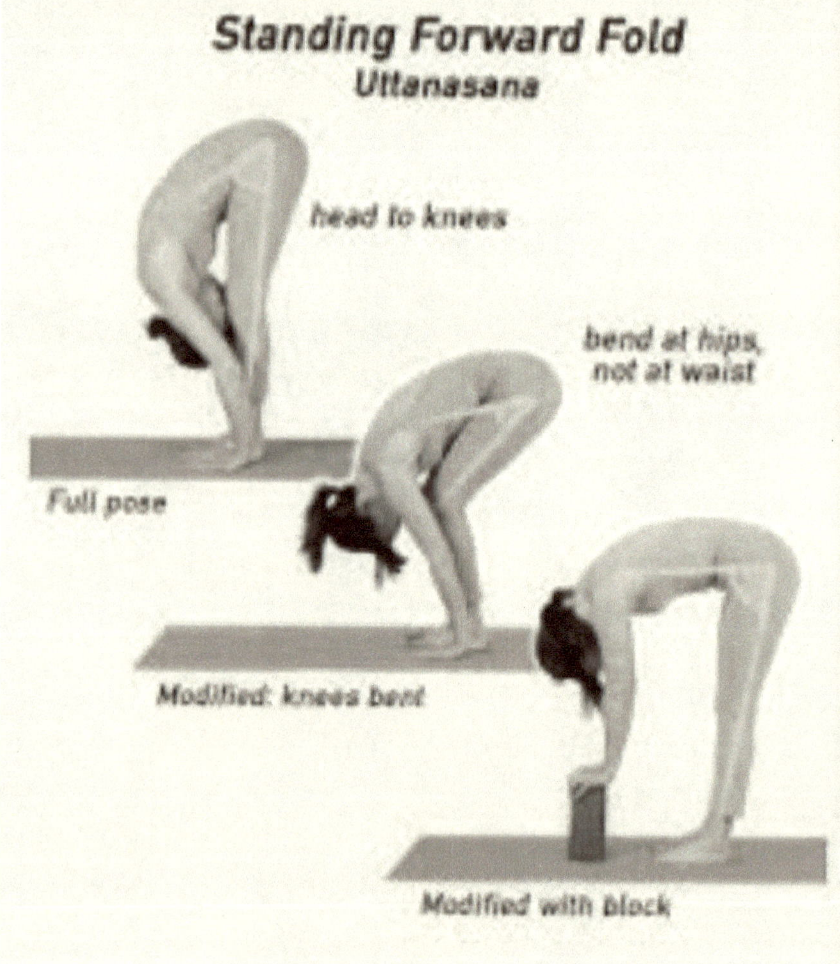

Remember, always listen to your body and work within your limits. If you have any concerns or medical conditions, please consult with a healthcare professional before attempting these poses. Regular practice of these balancing poses will not only improve your stability and coordination but also provide a sense of mindfulness and tranquility, making your journey as a silver yogi all the more fulfilling.

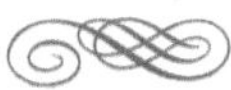

Strengthening Poses for Enhanced Muscular Health

AS WE AGE, IT BECOMES essential to focus on maintaining and enhancing our muscular health. Strong muscles not only help us perform daily activities with ease but also contribute to overall vitality and well-being. We will explore some strengthening poses designed for adults over 60, as part of our holistic approach to wellness through yoga.

Warrior II (Virabhadrasana):

This pose engages the legs, hips, and core, promoting leg strength and stability. Stand with your feet wide apart, extend your arms parallel to the floor, and bend your front knee while keeping your back leg straight. Hold the pose for a few breaths, feeling the strength build in your lower body.

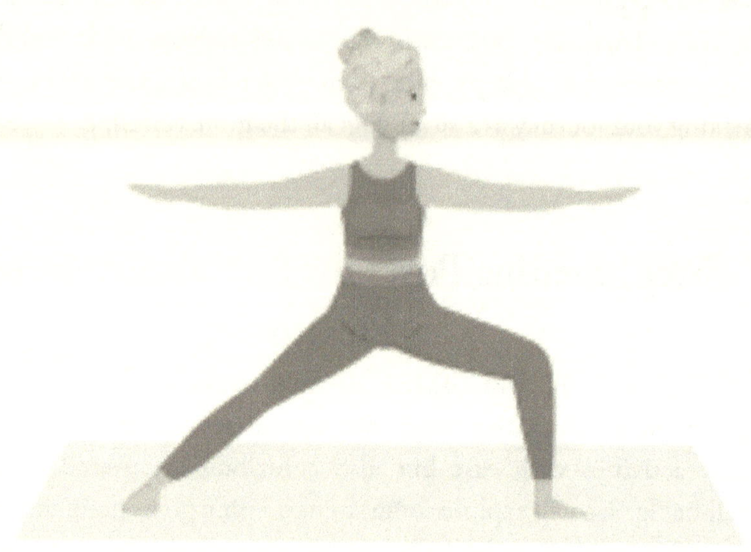

Warrior 2
Virabhadrasana II

Bridge pose (Setu Bandhasana):
This pose strengthens the glutes, hamstrings, and lower back. Lie on your back with knees bent, and feet flat on the floor. Inhale, lift your hips off the proud while pressing your feet into the floor, and interlace your hands underneath your back for support. Hold for several breaths, feeling the activation in your lower body.

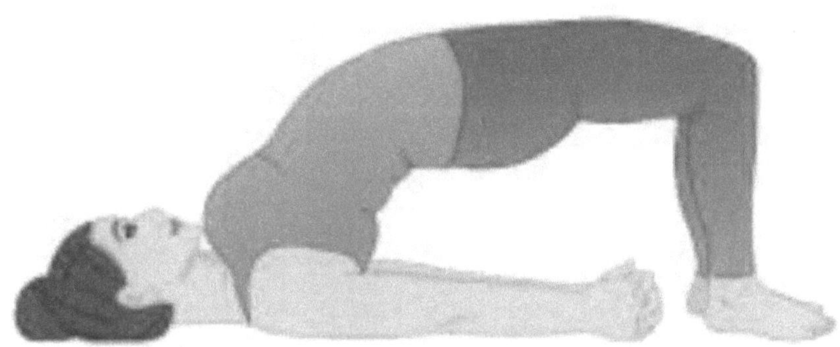

Chair pose (Utkatasana):

Chair pose is an excellent way to strengthen the legs and core. Stand with your feet hip-width apart, bend your knees, and lower yourself into an imaginary seated position. Extend your arms forward or upward for an added challenge. Stay in the pose for a few breaths, feeling your muscles working. You may hold onto a chair or place your back against the wall if needed for safety.

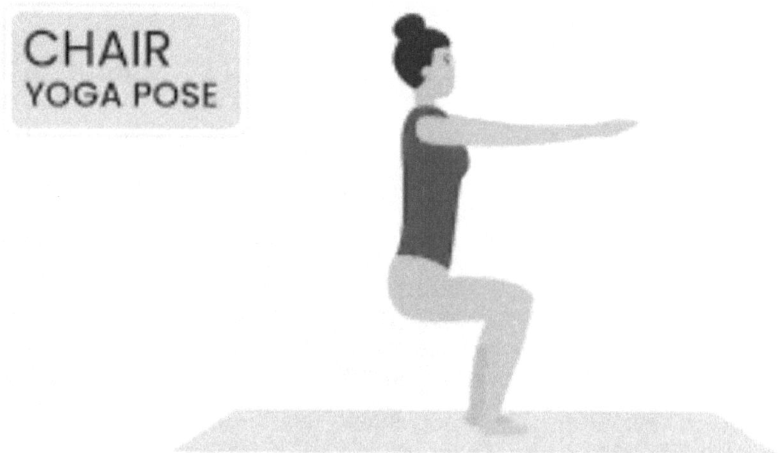

Tree pose (Vrikshasana):

This balancing pose targets the legs and improves stability. Stand tall and shift your weight onto one leg. Place your other foot on your inner thigh or calf., avoiding the knee joint. Find your balance and bring your hands together in a prayer position. You can use a chair to prop your knee on if needed. Hold for several breaths, then switch sides.

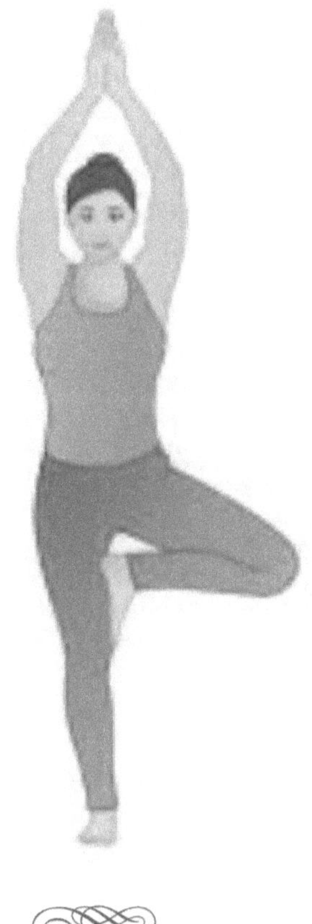

REMEMBER, EACH INDIVIDUAL'S fitness level may vary, so it's important to listen to your body and modify the poses as needed. Start slowly and gradually increase the duration and intensity of your practice. Regularly incorporating these strengthening poses into your yoga routine will help you maintain and enhance your muscular health, promoting a more active and fulfilling life.

Always consult with a healthcare professional before starting any new exercise program, especially if you have any pre-existing medical conditions. With dedication and consistency, yoga can be a transformative practice that supports your overall well-being, allowing you to thrive in your golden years.

Chapter Four:

Modifying Yoga Poses for Seniors

Using Props for Added Support and Comfort

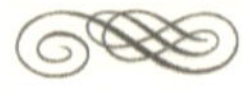

AS WE AGE, OUR BODIES change, and it is essential to adapt our yoga practice to accommodate these changes. Props can play a crucial role in providing the necessary support and comfort for seniors during their yoga sessions. Whether you are a beginner or have been practicing yoga for years, incorporating props into your routine can enhance your overall experience and make your practice more enjoyable.

Props such as blocks, straps, blankets, and bolsters can help seniors maintain proper alignment and prevent strain or injury. They provide stability and support, allowing individuals to hold poses for longer periods and explore deeper stretches. For those with limited flexibility or mobility, props can assist in achieving proper form and alignment, making yoga accessible to everyone.

Blocks are excellent tools for modifying postures and bringing the ground closer to you. They can be used to support your hands, feet, or hips, allowing for a more comfortable and stable foundation. Straps are beneficial for seniors with tight muscles or limited range of motion. They can be used to extend your reach, making it easier to grasp your feet or hold poses that require flexibility.

Blankets and bolsters are perfect for creating a soft and supportive surface during seated or lying poses. They provide cushioning for your joints and promote relaxation. Bolsters are especially useful for restorative poses, where they can be placed under the knees or lower back to release tension and promote deep relaxation.

Using props also allows seniors to modify poses to their comfort level, ensuring a safe and enjoyable practice. It is essential to listen to your body and use props as needed. Remember, yoga is not about perfection but about finding balance and harmony within yourself.

Incorporating props into your yoga practice can offer numerous benefits for seniors. They provide added support, enhance comfort, and allow for a more personalized and tailored experience. Props can help seniors maintain a consistent yoga practice, even if they have physical limitations or challenges.

So, whether you are new to yoga or have been practicing for years, don't hesitate to explore the world of props. Embrace them as valuable tools to enhance your practice and make it a truly holistic and rewarding experience.

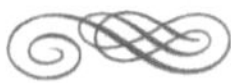

Adapting Poses for Limited Mobility or Chronic Conditions

AS WE AGE, WE COMMONLY experience decreased flexibility, mobility, and strength. However, we should not be discouraged from practicing yoga. In fact, yoga can be a wonderful tool for seniors to maintain and improve overall health and well-being. We will explore various ways to adapt yoga poses for individuals with limited mobility or chronic conditions.

Yoga is a versatile practice that can be modified to suit individual needs. For those with limited mobility, chair yoga is an excellent option. With the support of a chair, you can still experience the benefits of yoga without putting unnecessary strain on your joints. Seated poses such as the seated forward bend, seated twist, and seated side stretch can all be done with the aid of a chair. These poses help to stretch and strengthen the muscles while improving flexibility.

For individuals with chronic conditions such as arthritis or osteoporosis, it is important to approach yoga with caution and consult with a healthcare professional. Gentle poses such as the cat-cow stretch, gentle backbends, and standing forward bends can help alleviate stiffness and improve joint mobility. It is crucial to listen to your body and only go as far as feels comfortable. Remember, yoga is not about pushing yourself to the limit, but rather finding peace and harmony within your own body.

Props such as blocks, straps, and bolsters can be invaluable tools for adapting poses. A block or bolster can provide support and stability, making poses more accessible. Straps can assist with stretching and reaching. These props allow individuals with limited mobility to experience the benefits of yoga without compromising safety or comfort.

It is also important to practice mindfulness and self-compassion throughout your yoga journey. Each day is different, and it is okay to modify or skip certain poses based on how you feel. Remember that yoga is a personal practice, and the goal is not to achieve a perfect pose, but rather to honor and care for your body.

In conclusion, yoga is a powerful practice that can be adapted to suit individuals of all abilities and ages. By modifying poses and using props, seniors with limited mobility or chronic conditions can still experience the numerous benefits of yoga. Remember, to consult with a healthcare professional before starting any new exercise routine, and always listen to your body. Embrace the journey of yoga, and let it guide you toward holistic wellness and a renewed sense of vitality.

Practice Chair Yoga for Seated Modifications

As we age, it is important, that we stay active and maintain our physical and mental well-being. Yoga has proven to be an excellent practice for people of all ages, and seniors are no exception. In fact, yoga can be especially beneficial for older adults, helping to improve flexibility, strength, balance, and overall quality of life.

For adults over 60, chair yoga offers a safe and effective way to engage in this ancient practice. Chair yoga involves performing traditional yoga poses while seated or using a chair for support. This modification allows individuals with limited mobility or balance issues to experience the benefits of yoga.

One of the key advantages of chair yoga is that it can be done anywhere, making it accessible to seniors who may have difficulty getting to a yoga studio. All you need is a sturdy chair with no armrests, and you can create your own yoga space at home.

Chapter Five:

Breathing Techniques for Seniors

Deep Breathing Exercises for Stress Reduction

In today's fast-paced world, stress has become an inevitable part of our lives. The constant pressure, demands, and responsibilities can take a toll on our mental and physical well-being, especially for adults over 60. However, there is a powerful tool that can help seniors combat stress and achieve a state of calmness and tranquility with deep breathing exercises.

Deep breathing exercises are an integral part of yoga for seniors, as they provide numerous benefits for the mind, body, and spirit. By practicing these exercises regularly, older adults can reduce stress levels, improve their overall wellness, and enhance their quality of life.

One of the simplest deep breathing exercises for stress reduction is the 4-7-8 technique. Begin by finding a comfortable seated position, with your feet firmly planted on the ground and your spine straight. Close your eyes and take a deep breath in through your nose for a count of four. Hold your breath for a count of seven, and then exhale slowly through your mouth for a count of eight. Repeat this cycle three to four times, focusing on the sensation of your breath entering and leaving your body.

Another effective deep breathing exercise is alternative nostril breathing. Sit comfortably and use your right thumb to close your right nostril, while taking a deep breath in through your left nostril. Then, close your left nostril with your right ring finger and exhale through your right nostril. Inhale through your right nostril, close it with your thumb, and exhale through your left nostril. Repeat this process for several minutes, alternating the nostrils with each breath. This exercise helps balance the energy flow in your body, promoting relaxation and reducing stress.

By incorporating these deep breathing exercises into their daily routine, seniors can experience a wide range of benefits. Deep breathing triggers the body's relaxation response, lowering blood pressure, reducing muscle tension, and promoting a sense of calmness. It also improves lung function, enhances oxygenation of the blood, and boosts energy levels.

In conclusion, deep breathing exercises are a valuable tool for stress reduction in adults over 60. As part of the holistic wellness approach through yoga for seniors, these exercises can help older adults find inner peace, improve their well-being, and lead a more balanced life. So, take a moment each day to practice deep breathing and embrace the transformative power holds for your overall health and happiness.

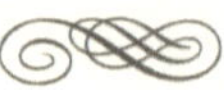

Pranayama Techniques for Improved Lung Function

AS WE AGE, IT IS NATURAL for our lung capacity to decrease, making it harder for us to take deep breaths and maintain optimal oxygen levels in our bodies. However, through the practice of pranayama, or yogic breathing exercises, we can significantly improve our lung function and enhance our overall well-being. We will explore some simple yet effective pranayama techniques specifically designed for seniors, to help you unlock the full potential of your lungs and promote holistic wellness.

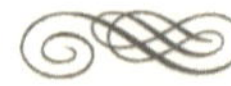

DEEP ABDOMINAL BREATHING:

One of the most fundamental pranayama techniques is deep abdominal breathing. Sit comfortably in a chair or on the floor, close your eyes, and place your hands on your abdomen. Inhale deeply through your nose, allowing your belly to expand as you fill your lungs with air. Exhale slowly through your mouth, emptying your lungs completely. Practice this technique for a few minutes each day to improve lung capacity and increase oxygen circulation throughout your body.

Alternate Nostril Breathing:

This technique helps balance the flow of energy in the body and enhances lung function. Sit in a comfortable position, close your eyes, and bring your right hand up to your face. Use your thumb to close your right nostril and inhale deeply through your left nostril. Now, close your left nostril with your ring finger and exhale through your right nostril. Repeat this pattern, alternating between nostrils, for several minutes. Alternate nostril breathing is known to calm the mind and improve lung efficiency.

Kapalabhati Breath:

This invigorating pranayama technique helps clear the respiratory system of toxins and promotes lung strength. Sit with your spine straight, close your eyes, and place your hands on your abdomen. Take a deep inhalation, and as you exhale forcefully through your nose, contract your abdominal muscles to expel the air. Allow your inhalations to happen naturally as your abdomen relaxes. Start with a few rounds and gradually increase the pace. This technique is not recommended for those with high blood pressure or heart conditions.

By incorporating these pranayama techniques into your daily routine, you can experience improved lung function and enjoy the many benefits of enhanced oxygenation. Remember, always listen to your body, start slowly, and consult a healthcare provider if you have any concerns. Embrace the power of pranayama and unlock your full potential as a silver yogi, achieving holistic wellness through yoga for seniors.

Energizing Breathwork for Mental Clarity and Focus

As we age, it is essential to prioritize our mental health and maintain a sharp focus. One powerful tool that can help us achieve this is breathwork. We will explore various breathwork techniques that are specifically tailored for seniors, allowing us to enhance our mental clarity and focus.

Breathwork is an integral aspect of yoga for seniors, as it helps us connect with our body and mind. By consciously controlling our breath, we can influence our state of mind and improve our overall well-being.

The following breathwork techniques are designed to invigorate and energize, promoting mental clarity and focus: Ujjayi Breath, Kapalabhati Breath, Alternate Nostril Breathing, and Bellows Breath.

Ujjayi Breath:

Also known as "victorious breath," this technique involves breathing in and out through the nose while slightly constricting the back of the throat. Ujjayi breath creates a gentle ocean-like sound and helps to calm the mind, reduce anxiety, and increase focus. Practice this breath during your yoga sessions or anytime you need to regain mental clarity.

Kapalabhati Breath:

This powerful breathwork technique involves rapid, forceful exhalations through the nose while keeping the inhalations passive. Kapalabhati breath helps to cleanse the mind, increase oxygen flow, and invigorate the body. Start with a few rounds of 10-20 breaths and gradually increase the duration as you feel comfortable.

Alternate Nostril Breathing:

This technique is excellent for balancing the left and right hemispheres of the brain, improving focus, and promoting mental clarity. Sit comfortably and use your right thumb to gently close your right nostril. Inhale deeply through the left nostril, then close it with your right ring finger and exhale through the right nostril. Repeat this cycle for a few minutes, alternating nostrils.

Bellows Breath:

Also known as Bhastrika, this breathwork technique involves forceful inhales and exhales through the nose while keeping a steady rhythm. Bellows breath increases oxygen intake, energizes the body, and enhances mental alertness. Begin with 10-15 breaths and gradually increase the intensity and duration over time.

Remember, breathwork is a powerful tool, but it's essential to listen to your body and never strain or force the breath. Find a comfortable seated position, preferably with a straight spine, and practice these breathwork techniques regularly to experience the benefit of enhanced mental clarity and focus.

Incorporating these energizing breathwork techniques into your daily routine will not only improve your mental clarity and focus but also provide a sense of calm and inner peace. Embrace the power of breathwork for a holistic approach to wellness as a senior yogi.

Chapter Six:

Mindfulness and Meditation for Seniors

Cultivating Mindfulness in Daily Life

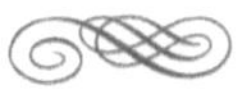

AS WE AGE, IT BECOMES even more essential to take care of our mental and emotional well-being. Cultivating mindfulness in our daily lives can greatly contribute to our overall sense of peace, happiness, and holistic wellness. We will explore how yoga can be a powerful tool in helping seniors cultivate mindfulness and bring a sense of tranquility to their daily routines.

Mindfulness is the practice of being fully present in the moment, without judgment or attachment. It allows us to become aware of our thoughts, emotions, and physical sensations, helping us better understand ourselves and navigate life's challenges with grace. Incorporating mindfulness into our daily lives can significantly enhance our quality of life.

Yoga, specifically tailored for seniors, offers a gentle yet effective way to cultivate mindfulness. Through a series of postures, breathwork, and meditation, seniors can learn to connect with their bodies, calm their minds, and find inner peace.

One of the key aspects of cultivating mindfulness in yoga is focusing on the breath. Deep, conscious breathing helps seniors become more present, calm their nervous system, and increase their mental clarity. The book includes various breathing exercises that can be practiced both on and off the yoga mat, allowing seniors to incorporate mindfulness into their daily lives.

Another important element of mindfulness is body awareness. Yoga postures, such as gentle stretches, balanced exercises, and seated poses, encourage seniors to pay attention to their bodies and their physical sensations. By mindfully moving through the postures, seniors can improve their flexibility, strength, and balance while also fostering a deep connection with their bodies.

In addition to the physical practice, the importance of meditation and mindfulness exercises must be emphasized. These practices help seniors develop a calm and focused mind, reduce stress, and enhance their overall well-being. This book provides simple meditation techniques that can be easily incorporated into daily routines, empowering seniors to find peace and stillness amidst the busyness of life.

By cultivating mindfulness in daily life through yoga, seniors can experience a profound transformation. They can develop a deeper sense of self-awareness, greater resilience in the face of challenges, and a renewed zest for life. The Silver Yogi serves as a comprehensive resource and guide, empowering adults over 60, to embrace yoga as a pathway to holistic wellness and enhanced mindfulness.

Practice Meditation for Relaxation and Mental Wellbeing

In the journey toward holistic wellness through yoga, meditation is an integral practice that can greatly benefit adults over 60. As we age, it becomes even more crucial to prioritize our mental well-being alongside our physical health. Meditation offers a powerful tool to cultivate inner peace, reduce stress, and enhance overall mental clarity.

Meditation is a practice of training the mind to focus on the present moment, allowing us to let go of unnecessary thoughts and worries. It can be done in various ways, such as focusing on the breath, repeating a mantra, or visualizing peaceful imagery. By engaging in regular meditation sessions, seniors can experience immense relaxation and find a sense of tranquility amidst the chaos of everyday life.

One of the primary benefits of meditation is stress reduction. As we age, life can become more demanding, filled with responsibilities, health challenges, and transitions. Meditation provides seniors with a refuge from external pressures and offers a chance to recharge and rejuvenate their minds. Research has shown that meditation can lower cortisol levels, the hormone responsible for stress, and improve overall mental resilience.

Furthermore, meditation also helps improve concentration and memory retention, which can be particularly valuable for seniors. By training the mind to focus and be present, meditation enhances cognitive function and mental agility. It can help seniors maintain sharpness and mental clarity, allowing them to navigate daily tasks with ease.

Moreover, meditation has been linked to a decrease in anxiety and depression symptoms. The practice helps calm the mind, creating a sense of inner peace and contentment. By incorporating meditation into their daily routine, seniors can find solace in the present moment and develop a positive outlook toward life.

To begin practicing meditation, find a quiet and comfortable spot where you can sit or lie down. Close your eyes, take deep breaths, and let go of any tension in your body. Focus on your breath, feeling the sensation of each inhale and exhale. As thoughts arise, gently let go and redirect your attention to your breath. Start with shorter sessions and gradually increase the duration as you become more comfortable.

Remember, meditation is a personal journey, and it may take time to reap its full benefits. Be patient and compassionate with yourself as you embark on this transformative practice. With regular meditation, seniors can unlock a profound sense of relaxation, mental well-being, and inner peace.

Incorporating Mindfulness into Yoga Practice

As we gracefully age, it becomes increasingly important to prioritize our overall well-being, and one practice that has proven to be immensely beneficial for adults over 60 is yoga. However, to truly unlock the transformative power of this ancient discipline, it is essential to incorporate mindfulness into our yoga practice.

Mindfulness is the art of being present in the moment, fully aware of our thoughts, feelings, and sensations without judgment. It allows us to cultivate a deep sense of self-awareness and harnesses the power of our minds to enhance our yoga practice, both on and off the mat.

When we incorporate mindfulness into our yoga practice, we create an opportunity to connect with our bodies, cultivate gratitude for the present moment, and develop a sense of compassion toward ourselves. This is particularly crucial for seniors as it helps foster a positive mindset and promotes a greater understanding of our bodies' unique needs and limitations.

To begin incorporating mindfulness into your yoga practice, start by selling an intention before each session. This can be as simple as dedicating the practice to self-care or focusing on gratitude for your body's ability to move and stretch. Take a few moments to quiet your mind, center yourself, and bring awareness to your breath.

During your yoga practice, pay close attention to the sensations in your body. Notice any areas of tension or discomfort and adjust your poses accordingly. Mindfully move through each asana, focusing on the alignment of your body and the gentle flow of your breath. Allow yourself to fully experience the present moment, surrendering any thoughts or distractions that may arise.

As you move through your yoga practice, be kind and compassionate toward yourself. Embrace the notion that everybody is unique and that your practice is about honoring your own journey. Avoid comparing yourself to others and instead celebrate your progress, no matter how small.

Beyond the physical benefits, incorporating mindfulness into your yoga practice can have profound effects on your mental and emotional well-being. It can reduce stress, anxiety, and depression while increasing feelings of calmness, clarity, and overall happiness.

In conclusion, as adults over 60, we have the power to enhance our yoga practice by incorporating mindfulness. By setting intentions, being present, and practicing self-compassion, we can deepen our connection with our bodies, find joy in the present moment, and cultivate a greater sense of well-being. Embrace mindfulness as an essential tool on your yoga journey and unlock the transformative power it holds for your body, mind, and spirit.

Chapter Seven:

Embracing Yoga as a Lifestyle for Seniors

Integrating Yoga Philosophy into Daily Activities

Yoga is not just about physical exercises and poses; it is a holistic way of life that encompasses mind, body, and spirit. For adults over 60 who are seeking to enhance their overall well-being, incorporating yoga philosophy into daily activities can be transformative. We will explore how seniors can seamlessly integrate the principles of yoga into their everyday lives, leading to a more balanced and fulfilling existence.

Mindfulness in Every Moment:

One of the core tenets of yoga philosophy is mindfulness - being fully present in the moment. Seniors can practice mindfulness in their daily activities by consciously focusing on each task, whether it is cooking, gardening, or even walking. By bringing awareness to their actions, seniors can experience a deeper sense of connection with themselves and their surroundings.

Breathing Exercises:

The breath is a powerful tool in yoga, and seniors can utilize specific breathing exercises to promote relaxation and reduce anxiety. By incorporating deep, conscious breathing into their daily routines, seniors can enhance their overall well-being and cultivate a sense of calm and tranquility.

Gratitude Practice:

Gratitude is an essential aspect of yoga philosophy, and seniors can cultivate this through a daily gratitude practice. Taking a few moments each day to reflect on the things that are grateful for can shift their focus from negativity to positivity, leading to a more joyful and contented outlook on life.

Yoga Inspired Stretching:

Seniors can infuse their daily activities with yoga-inspired stretching exercises. Whether it is gentle stretches while watching television, incorporating yoga poses into household chores, or watching television, incorporating yoga poses into household chores, or taking breaks throughout the day to stretch and release tension, these activities can improve flexibility, joint mobility, and overall physical well-being.

Self-care Rituals:

Yoga philosophy emphasizes self-care and self-love. Seniors can honor their bodies and minds by incorporating self-care rituals into their daily routines. This may include taking regular baths with soothing essential oils, practicing gentle self-massage, or dedicating time to rest and relax.

Integrating yoga philosophy into daily activities is a powerful way for seniors to enhance their overall well-being and find harmony in their lives. By embracing mindfulness, gratitude, breathing exercises, stretching, and self-care, seniors can experience the transformative benefits of yoga on a daily basis.

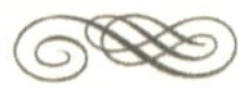

Nurturing Emotional Wellbeing through Yoga

AS WE AGE, IT BECOMES increasingly important to prioritize our emotional well-being. The ups and downs of life can take a toll on our mental health if we don't actively take steps to nurture it. One powerful tool that we can support the emotional well-being of seniors is yoga. We will explore how yoga can enhance emotional health and provide practical tips for incorporating it into your daily routine.

Yoga is a holistic practice that connects the mind, body, and spirit. It offers a range of benefits for seniors, including flexibility, balance, and strength. However, its impact on emotional well-being should not be overlooked. Regular yoga practice has been shown to reduce stress, anxiety, and depression, all common emotional challenges that many seniors face.

One of the key ways yoga supports emotional well-being is by promoting mindfulness. Mindfulness is the practice of being fully present in the current moment, without judgment. Through various yoga poses, breathing exercises, and meditation techniques, seniors can cultivate mindfulness and develop a deeper connection with their emotions. This heightened awareness allows them to better understand their feelings, manage stress, and respond to challenging situations with greater resilience.

Additionally, yoga provides a safe space for seniors to express and release emotions. The gentle movements and stretches in yoga poses can help release tension from the body, creating a sense of emotional release as well. By creating an environment of self-acceptance and self-care, yoga encourages seniors to explore their emotions and embrace them without judgment.

To incorporate yoga into your daily routine, start with simple and gentle poses that are suitable for your body and ability level. It's important to listen to your body and never push yourself beyond your limits. Attending senior-specific yoga classes or working with a qualified yoga instructor who specializes in yoga for seniors can provide guidance and ensure proper alignment to prevent injuries.

Remember, emotional well-being is just as important as physical health in the journey of aging gracefully. By nurturing your emotional health through yoga, you can find a sense of peace, balance, and joy in your golden years. So, roll out your yoga mat, take a deep breath, and embark on this transformative journey toward holistic wellness.

Creating a Personalized Yoga Routine for Long-Term Wellness

As adults over 60, it is essential to prioritize our overall well-being and maintain a healthy lifestyle. One powerful way to achieve this is through the practice of yoga. Yoga for seniors can have remarkable benefits, including increased flexibility, improved balance, enhanced mental, clarity, reduced stress, and a stronger sense of overall well-being. We will explore the process of creating a personalized yoga routine specifically tailored to meet your unique needs and goals for long-term wellness.

Before diving into the specifics of creating a personalized yoga routine, it is important to consult with a qualified yoga instructor or healthcare professional. They can assess your current physical condition and provide guidance on any modifications for precautions you may need to take based on your individual circumstances.

The first step in creating a personalized yoga routine is to identify your goals. Are you looking to improve flexibility, build strength, reduce stress, or address specific health concerns? Once you have a clear understanding of your objectives, you can select yoga poses and sequences that align with your goals.

Next, consider your physical condition and any limitations you may have. It's crucial to listen to your body and choose poses that are safe and comfortable for you. Yoga is a highly adaptable practice, and there are modifications available for almost every pose to accommodate various abilities and needs.

As you begin to design your routine, aim for a balanced combination of poses that target different areas of the body. Include standing poses for strength and stability, seated poses for flexibility and mobility, and gentle inversions for improved circulation. Incorporating breathing exercises and meditation into your routine can also nurture mental clarity and promote relaxation.

Remember to start slowly and gradually increase the intensity and duration of your practice. It's important to give your body time to adapt and avoid overexertion or injury. Consistency is key; aim for regular practice, even if it's just a few minutes each day, to experience the long-term benefits of yoga.

Lastly, be open to exploring different styles and approaches to yoga. There is no one-size-fits-all approach, and what works for one person may not work for another. Allow yourself the freedom to experiment and find the routines and poses that resonate with you on a personal level.

By creating a personalized yoga routine for long-term wellness, you are investing in your physical, mental, and emotional well-being. Embrace the journey, enjoy the practice, and witness the transformative power of yoga in your life.

Chapter Eight:

Yoga for Specific Health Concerns in Seniors

Managing Arthritis and Joint Pain through Yoga

As we age, our bodies go through various changes, and one common challenge faced by many older adults is arthritis and joint pain. The good news is that yoga, a gentle and holistic practice, can provide immense relief and help manage these conditions effectively. We will explore how yoga can be an invaluable tool for adults over 60 in overcoming arthritis and joint pain, allowing them to lead a more active and pain-free life.

Yoga offers numerous benefits for seniors, including increased flexibility, improved balance, enhanced strength, and reduced stress. These benefits are particularly advantageous for individuals dealing with arthritis and joint pain. Through a combination of gentle movements, stretches, and breathing exercises, yoga helps to alleviate stiffness, reduce inflammation, and improve joint mobility.

The practice of yoga encourages mindfulness and self-awareness, allowing seniors to tune in to their bodies and make mindful choices that support their health and well-being. By listening to their bodies and practicing yoga mindfully, seniors can avoid overexertion or strain, ensuring a safe and effective practice.

Specific yoga poses and sequences can target areas commonly affected by arthritis and joint pain, such as the knees, hips, and hands. Poses like Cat-Cow, Child's Pose, and Gentle Seated Twist can help increase flexibility and relieve tension in the spine. Modified versions of classic poses like Downward-Facing Dog and Warrior II can be practiced with the support of props, making them accessible to seniors with joint pain.

Additionally, breathing exercises, such as Deep Belly Breathing and Alternate Nostril Breathing, can be incorporated into the yoga practice to promote relaxation and reduce stress, which can further alleviate pain and inflammation.

It is important to note that seniors should always consult their healthcare provider before starting a new exercise regimen, including yoga. Working with a qualified yoga instructor experienced in teaching yoga to seniors is also highly recommended to ensure proper guidance and modifications tailored to individual needs.

By incorporating yoga into their daily routine, seniors can manage arthritis and joint pain naturally, without relying solely on medication. Yoga helps seniors improve their overall well-being and enjoy a pain-free, active lifestyle in their golden years. Remember, it is never too late to start practicing yoga, and with dedication and consistency, its transformative benefits can be experienced by every adult over 60.

Promoting Heart Health and Circulation with Yoga

As we age, it becomes increasingly important to prioritize our heart health and circulation. Yoga, with its gentle yet effective movements and breathing techniques, is an ideal practice for seniors looking to maintain a healthy heart and improve blood flow throughout the body.

Yoga offers numerous benefits for adults over 60, specifically targeting heart health and circulation. The practice helps reduce blood pressure, lowers heart rate, and improves overall cardiovascular fitness. By engaging in regular yoga sessions, seniors can enhance their heart's efficiency, strengthen the cardiovascular system, and reduce the risk of heart-related diseases.

One of the key aspects of yoga that promotes heart health is its emphasis on deep, mindful breathing. Pranayama, or yogic breathing exercises, help seniors expand their lung capacity, increase oxygen intake, and enhance blood oxygenation. This results in improved circulation, as oxygen-rich blood is pumped more efficiently to vital organs, muscles, and tissues. Additionally, pranayama techniques such as alternate nostril breathing and deep belly breathing help calm the mind, reduce stress, and balance the autonomic nervous system, further benefiting heart health.

Yoga asanas, or postures, also play a pivotal role in promoting heart health and circulation. Gentle poses like mountain pose, seated forward bend, and bridge pose help stretch and strengthen the muscles, including the heart. These poses stimulate blood flow, improve flexibility, and provide a low-impact workout for seniors, ensuring their hearts remain healthy and active.

Furthermore, practicing yoga can aid in weight management, another crucial factor in maintaining heart health. Regular yoga sessions, combined with a balanced diet, can help seniors achieve and maintain a healthy weight, reducing the strain on the heart and blood vessels. By shedding excess pounds, seniors can significantly lower the risk of heart disease, high cholesterol, and other cardiovascular conditions.

In conclusion, yoga is a powerful tool for promoting heart health and circulation in adults over 60. Through its combination of gentle movements, breathing exercises, and relaxation techniques, yoga provides a holistic approach to maintaining cardiovascular fitness. By incorporating yoga into their daily routine, seniors can enhance their heart's function, improve blood flow, and enjoy a healthier, more active lifestyle. Remember, it's never too late to start practicing yoga and reap its numerous benefits for the heart and overall well-being.

Enhancing Bone Density and Preventing Osteoporosis

As we age, maintaining strong bones becomes increasingly important. Osteoporosis, a condition characterized by weak and brittle bones, affects millions of adults over the age of 60. However, there are numerous ways to enhance bone density and prevent the onset of osteoporosis, and practicing yoga is a powerful tool in achieving this goal.

Yoga for seniors is a gentle and effective practice that can significantly contribute to bone health. The weight-bearing nature of many yoga poses stimulates the bones, encouraging them to become stronger and denser. Additionally, yoga helps improve balance and coordination, reducing the risk of falls and fractures, which is especially crucial for individuals with osteoporosis.

One of the key benefits of yoga for bone health is its ability to promote flexibility and range of motion. By regularly practicing yoga, seniors can maintain joint mobility, preventing stiffness and reducing the risk of fractures caused by falls. Gentle stretches and movements in yoga poses also help to strengthen the muscles surrounding the bones, providing additional support and stability.

Certain yoga poses are particularly beneficial for enhancing bone density and preventing osteoporosis. Poses such as Warrior II, Triangle, and Tree pose help to strengthen the hips, legs, and spine, which are common areas of concern for individuals with osteoporosis. These poses also engage the core muscles, promoting better posture and balance.

In addition to physical postures, breathing exercises, and meditation techniques incorporated in yoga can help seniors manage stress. Chronic stress has been linked to a decrease in bone density, so by reducing stress levels through yoga, we can indirectly contribute to the overall health of our bones.

It is essential for seniors to practice yoga under the guidance of a qualified instructor who specializes in yoga for seniors. They can provide modifications and adaptations to ensure safety and tailor the practice to individual needs and abilities. It is also advisable to consult with a healthcare professional before starting any new exercise regimen, especially if you have a pre-existing condition or are taking medication.

By embracing yoga as part of your daily routine, you can enhance bone density, prevent osteoporosis, and promote overall well-being. So, roll out your mat, take a deep breath, and embark on a journey toward holistic wellness through yoga for seniors. Your bones will thank you!

Chapter Nine:

Yoga for Brain Health and Cognitive Function

Improving Memory and Focus through Yoga

As we age, memory loss and a decline in cognitive function can often be a cause for concern. However, there is good news for seniors looking to enhance their mental abilities. Yoga can be a powerful tool for improving memory and focus. We will explore the various ways in which yoga can benefit the aging brain and provide practical exercises to help seniors maintain sharp minds.

Yoga is not just a physical practice; it encompasses a holistic approach to wellness. The combination of physical postures (asanas), breathing exercises (pranayama), and meditation can have a profound impact on the brain's cognitive functions. Regular yoga practice has been shown to increase blood flow to the brain, stimulate the growth of neural connections, and improve overall mental clarity.

One of the key benefits of yoga for seniors is stress reduction. Chronic stress can negatively affect memory and concentration. By incorporating relaxation techniques such as deep breathing and guided meditation into their yoga practice, seniors can learn to manage stress effectively. This, in turn, helps to improve memory and focus.

Certain yoga poses are particularly beneficial for enhancing cognitive function. Poses that require balance, such as the Tree Pose or the Eagle Pose, help improve focus and concentration. Inversions like Downward-Facing Dog or the Shoulder Stand increase blood flow to the brain, providing a refreshing boost of energy and clarity. Additionally, seated forward bends like the seated forward fold or the head-to-knee pose can calm the mind and improve memory.

Breathing exercises, or pranayama, can also play a crucial role in enhancing memory and focus. Techniques like alternate nostril breathing or the victorious breath can help regulate the flow of prana (life force energy) in the body, promoting mental clarity and sharpening cognitive abilities.

To make the most of yoga for memory improvement, consistency is key. Seniors over 60 should aim for regular practice, ideally three to five times per week. Starting gentle yoga classes specifically designed for seniors can be a great way to ease into the practice and gradually build strength and flexibility.

In conclusion, yoga provides a holistic approach to improving memory and focus in seniors over 60. By incorporating physical postures, breathing exercises, and meditation into their routine, seniors can enhance cognitive function, reduce stress levels, and sharpen their mental abilities. With regular practice, seniors can embark on a journey of holistic wellness, reaping the numerous benefits that yoga has to offer.

Enhancing Brain Plasticity and Neurological Health

As we age, it is natural for our bodies and minds to undergo certain changes. However, contrary to popular belief, cognitive decline and neurological issues are not inevitable as we grow older. In fact, there are several ways we can enhance brain plasticity and maintain neurological health well into our golden years. One such method that has proven to be highly effective is the practice of yoga for seniors.

Yoga, a holistic discipline that combines physical postures, breathing exercises, and meditation, offers a multitude of benefits for the aging population. Studies have shown that regular yoga practice can significantly improve brain plasticity, which refers to the brain's ability to adapt and reorganize itself throughout life. By engaging in yoga, seniors can stimulate their brains, create new neural connections, and enhance cognitive function.

One of the primary factors contributing to brain plasticity is physical activity. Yoga promotes gentle movement, stretching, and balance, which not only improve physical fitness but also enhance blood circulation to the brain. Increased blood flow delivers essential nutrients and oxygen, nourishing the brain and supporting its overall health. Moreover, yoga postures that involve balance and coordination help seniors maintain their proprioception, a key aspect of neurological health that allows us to sense our body's position in space.

In addition to the physical benefits, yoga also has a profound impact on mental and emotional well-being. Regular practice of meditation and breathing exercises can reduce stress and anxiety, which are known to have detrimental effects on brain health. By calming the mind and reducing mental clutter, yoga promotes a sense of clarity and focus, allowing seniors to better retain information and improve memory.

Furthermore, yoga offers a unique opportunity for seniors to engage in a social and supportive community, which plays a crucial role in maintaining neurological health. Participating in group yoga classes not only provides a sense of belonging but also stimulates social interactions and cognitive engagement, both of which have been linked to improved brain function.

Incorporating yoga into your daily routine can have a profound impact on brain plasticity and neurological health. Whether you are a seasoned yogi or new to the practice, it is never too late to start reaping the benefits of yoga for seniors. So roll out your mat, take a deep breath, and embark on a journey toward holistic wellness and a sharp mind.

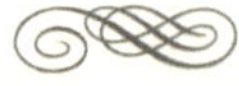

Combating Age-Related Cognitive Decline with Yoga

AS WE AGE, IT'S NATURAL for cognitive decline to become a concern. Many adults over 60 experience changes in memory, attention, and overall cognitive function. However, there is growing evidence to suggest that practicing yoga can help combat age-related cognitive decline and promote overall brain health.

Yoga is a holistic practice that combines physical postures, breathing exercises, and meditation. It has been practiced for thousands of years and is known to have a multitude of benefits for the mind, body, and spirit. When it comes to cognitive health, yoga offers a unique set of tools that can be particularly beneficial for seniors.

One of the key ways that yoga combats age-related cognitive decline is by reducing stress. Chronic stress has been linked to cognitive impairments, including memory loss and decreased attention span. By practicing yoga regularly, adults over 60 can lower their stress levels and promote a sense of calm and relaxation. This, in turn, can help improve cognitive function and enhance overall well-being.

Additionally, yoga improves blood circulation throughout the body, including the brain. This increased blood flow delivers essential nutrients and oxygen to the brain, aiding in its overall health and function. Studies have shown that regular yoga practice can improve cognitive performance, including memory, attention, and processing speed.

Moreover, yoga incorporates mindfulness and meditation practices, which have been shown to enhance cognitive function. Mindfulness involves paying attention to the present moment without judgment, allowing individuals to cultivate increased awareness and focus. By incorporating mindfulness into yoga practice, seniors can sharpen their cognitive skills and enhance their overall mental clarity.

Furthermore, yoga can also help improve sleep quality, which is essential for cognitive health. Many older adults struggle with insomnia or poor sleep, which can negatively impact memory and cognitive function. By practicing yoga regularly, individuals can experience better sleep, leading to improved cognitive performance and overall well-being.

In conclusion, yoga offers a multitude of benefits for seniors, including combating age-related cognitive decline. By reducing stress, improving blood circulation, promoting mindfulness, and enhancing sleep quality, yoga can help seniors maintain and improve their cognitive function. Incorporating yoga into daily life can lead to a sharper mind, improved memory, and overall holistic wellness. So, if you're an adult over 60, it's never too late to start your yoga journey and unlock the potential for a healthier, more vibrant mind.

Chapter Ten:

Holistic Lifestyle Tips for Seniors

Nutrition and Diet Recommendations for Optimal Wellness

As we age, maintaining optimal wellness becomes increasingly important. One of the key aspects of achieving this is through a balanced and nutritious diet. We will explore the nutrition and diet recommendations specifically tailored for seniors practicing yoga to enhance their overall well-being.

As adults over 60, our bodies undergo various physiological changes that can affect our nutritional needs. It is crucial to focus on consuming nutrient-dense foods that provide essential vitamins, minerals, and antioxidants. These nutrients help support our immune system, prevent chronic diseases, and promote healthy aging.

First and foremost, hydration is vital. Seniors are more susceptible to dehydration, so it is essential to drink plenty of water throughout the day. Hydration supports joint health, digestion, and overall bodily functions, allowing us to fully engage in our yoga practice and daily activities.

Next, a well-balanced diet should include a variety of fruits and vegetables. These colorful foods are packed with fiber, vitamins, and minerals. Aim to consume at least five servings of fruit and vegetables daily, incorporating a rainbow of options to ensure a wide range of nutrients. Additionally, whole grains such as quinoa, brown rice, and whole wheat bread provide sustained energy and are excellent sources of dietary fiber.

Protein consumption is also crucial for seniors practicing yoga. Lean meats, fish, eggs, dairy products, and plant-based sources like beans, lentils, and tofu are excellent choices. Protein aids muscle recovery, strengthens bones, and supports overall strength and mobility.

Furthermore, healthy fats play a vital role in our well-being. Incorporate sources like avocados, nuts, seeds, and olive oil into your diet. These fats provide essential fatty acids that support brain health, reduce inflammation, and improve heart health.

Lastly, it is important to be mindful of portion sizes. As our metabolism slows down with age, it is easier to consume excess calories, leading to weight gain. Practice portion control and listen to your body's hunger and fullness cues.

Remember, nutrition is only one piece of the puzzle. Combine these dietary recommendations with regular yoga practice to achieve optimal wellness. By nourishing your body with nutrient-dense foods and staying hydrated, you will enhance your yoga practice, promote healthy aging, and enjoy a vibrant and fulfilling life.

In conclusion, prioritizing nutrition and diet is fundamental for adults over 60 practicing yoga. By following these recommendations and incorporating them into your daily life, you will pave the way for optimal wellness, allowing you to embrace the benefits of yoga for seniors fully.

Sleep and Relaxation Techniques for Restorative Rest

As we age, it becomes increasingly important to our sleep and relaxation in order to maintain our overall health and well-being. Lack of quality sleep can lead to a range of issues, including increased stress levels, decreased cognitive function, and a weakened immune system. We will explore various sleep and relaxation techniques specifically designed for seniors, with a focus on incorporating yoga into our daily routines.

Yoga has long been recognized as an effective practice for promoting relaxation and restful sleep. The gentle, low-impact nature of yoga makes it an ideal exercise for seniors, as it can be easily modified to accommodate different fitness levels and physical abilities. By incorporating yoga into our daily lives, we can reap the benefits of improved sleep and overall well-being.

One of the key principles of yoga for seniors is the emphasis on deep breathing and mindfulness. Deep breathing exercises, such as the "4-7-8" technique, can help calm the mind and relax the body, preparing us for a restful night's sleep. By taking slow, deep breaths and focusing on the present moment, we can quiet our thoughts and release tension from our bodies.

In addition to deep breathing, gentle stretching, and relaxation poses can also aid in promoting restorative rest. Poses such as Child's Pose, Legs-Up-The-Wall, and Corpse Pose can help release tension from the body and promote relaxation. These poses can be practiced before bed or as part of a bedtime routine to signal to the body that it's time to wind down and prepare for sleep.

Creating a comfortable sleep environment is also crucial for restorative rest. Investing in a supportive mattress and pillows, ensuring a dark and quiet room, and implementing a consistent bedtime routine can all contribute to a better night's sleep for seniors. Additionally, avoiding stimulating activities, such as watching TV or using electronic devices, before bed can help promote relaxation and improve sleep quality.

By incorporating these sleep and relaxation techniques into our daily routines, we can experience the benefits of restorative rest and improve our overall well-being. Remember, it's never too late to prioritize our sleep and take steps toward a healthier, more rejuvenated lifestyle.

Social Connection and Building a Supportive Community

As we age, maintaining social connections becomes increasingly important for our overall well-being. The power of social connection should never be underestimated, as it plays a vital role in promoting good mental, emotional, and physical health. We will explore the significance of social connections for adults over 60 and how yoga can help foster these connections, ultimately building a supportive community.

As we transition into our golden years, life can sometimes feel isolating. Friends and family may have moved away, and the loss of loved ones becomes more frequent. However, it is essential to remember that we are not alone. There are countless individuals in similar situations, seeking companionship and understanding. Yoga for seniors provides a unique opportunity to connect with others who share similar interests and experiences.

Joining a yoga class specifically designed for seniors can be an excellent way to meet new people and build lasting friendships. These classes provide a safe and welcoming environment where individuals can chrome together, learn, and grow. The sense of community that develops within these yoga classes is invaluable, as it offers a support system that extends beyond the mat.

Engaging in yoga, breathing exercises, and meditation alongside fellow seniors can foster a sense of camaraderie and understanding. Sharing stories, laughter, and challenges during these sessions allows for genuine connections to form and helps combat feelings of loneliness and isolation. These connections often extend beyond the yoga studio, as participants may choose to socialize and bond outside of class as well.

Being part of a supportive community not only enhances our social well-being but also positively impacts our overall health. Research has shown that social connections can help reduce the risk of chronic diseases, improve cognitive function, boost immune system function, and increase longevity. Additionally, having a strong support system can provide emotional comfort during challenging times and promote a positive outlook on life.

In conclusion, social connection and building a supportive community are vital aspects of holistic wellness for adults over 60. Engaging in yoga for seniors offers a unique opportunity to connect with others, share experiences, and build lasting friendships. By joining a yoga class designed specifically for seniors, individuals can foster a sense of community and combat feelings of isolation, ultimately improving their overall well-being. So, take the first step toward building a supportive community, and discover the transformative power of yoga for seniors.

Chapter Eleven

Overcoming Barriers and Motivating Seniors in Yoga Practice

Addressing Common Concerns and Fears About Yoga

As adults over 60, it is perfectly natural to have concerns and fears about starting a new exercise routine, especially when it comes to something as unfamiliar as yoga. However, it is important to understand that yoga is a gentle and holistic practice that can greatly benefit seniors in numerous ways. Let's address some of the common concerns and fears about yoga for seniors, and hopefully ease your mind about embarking on this wonderful journey toward holistic wellness.

One of the most common concerns is the fear of injury. Many seniors worry that they may not be flexible enough or that they might strain a muscle while attempting yoga poses. It is important to remember that yoga is a practice that can be modified to suit individual needs and abilities. A qualified instructor who specializes in yoga for seniors will be able to guide you through the poses, ensuring that you are practicing safely and effectively.

Another concern is the fear of feeling out of place or uncomfortable in a yoga class. It is normal to feel self-conscious when trying something new, but rest assured, yoga classes for seniors are designed to create a welcoming and supportive environment. You will be surrounded by like-minded individuals who share similar goals of improving their overall well-being. It's a great opportunity to meet new people and make lasting connections.

Some seniors worry about their ability to keep up with the pace of a yoga class. It's important to remember that yoga is not a competitive sport. It is a personal practice that allows you to move at your own pace. In fact, yoga encourages you to listen to your body, honor its limitations, and work within your own comfort zone. With regular practice, you will gradually build strength, flexibility, and balance.

Lastly, there may be concerns about the spiritual aspect of yoga. While yoga originated as a spiritual practice, it has evolved over the years to cater to a wide range of individuals, including those who may not be interested in the spiritual aspects. Yoga for seniors is often focused on physical postures, breathing exercises, and relaxation techniques, which can all be enjoyed without delving into the spiritual realm.

In conclusion, it is completely normal to have concerns and fears about starting yoga as a senior. However, addressing these concerns and fears can help you overcome any hesitations and embrace the numerous benefits that yoga can offer. Remember, yoga is a gentle and adaptable practice that can be tailored to suit your individual needs and abilities. So, take that first step, join a yoga class for seniors, and embark on a journey toward holistic wellness and improved well-being.

Encouraging Consistency and Self-Motivation in Yoga

In the journey toward holistic wellness through yoga, consistency, and self-motivation play vital roles, especially for seniors. As adults over 60, it is essential to embrace these qualities to reap the full benefits that yoga offers. Here we will guide you on how to cultivate consistency and self-motivation in your yoga practice, empowering you to maintain a vibrant and fulfilling lifestyle.

Consistency is the key to progress in any endeavor, and yoga is no exception. By setting a regular schedule for your practice, you create a sense of discipline and commitment. Dedicate specific times of the day or week to your yoga sessions, making it a non-negotiable part of your routine. Consider finding a comfortable space at home or joining a local yoga class that caters to seniors. Having a designated area and a supportive community will enhance your motivation and make it easier to stick to your practice.

To encourage consistency, it is crucial to set realistic goals. Start with attainable adjectives, such as attending two yoga sessions per week or mastering a particular pose within a certain timeframe. Celebrate each milestone achieved, and gradually increase the difficulty level as you progress. Remember, yoga is a personal journey, and comparing yourself to others can hinder your motivation. Embrace your unique pace and focus on your own growth.

Self-motivation is the driving force behind consistent yoga practice. Understanding the transformative power of yoga can serve as a powerful motivator. Reflect on the positive changes you have experienced in terms of physical strength, flexibility, mental clarity, and emotional well-being. Maintains a journal to track your progress, noting both physical and mental improvements. This practice will remind you of the incredible impact yoga has on your overall wellness, motivating you to continue and explore new horizons.

Moreover, finding joy in your yoga practice is essential. Experiment with different styles of yoga and explore various poses to discover what resonates with you the most. Incorporate elements of mindfulness and meditation, allowing yourself to connect with your inner self during your practice. Engage in positive self-talk, reminding yourself of the incredible capabilities of your body and mind. Surrounding yourself with like-minded individuals who share your passion for yoga, exchanging experiences, and supporting each other along the way.

In conclusion, consistency and self-motivation are the pillars of a successful yoga practice, especially for seniors. Embrace a regular schedule, set realistic goals, and celebrate your achievements. Reflect on the transformative power of yoga and find joy in your practice. By cultivating these qualities, you can unlock the full potential of yoga, leading to holistic wellness and a fulfilling life as a silver yogi.

Chapter Twelve:

Taking Yoga Beyond the Mat for Seniors

Incorporating Yoga Principles into Daily Life Activities

As we age, it becomes increasingly important to maintain a healthy and active lifestyle. Yoga offers a multitude of benefits for seniors, including improved flexibility, strength, balance, and mental well-being. However, the benefits of yoga extend far beyond the mat and can be incorporated into our daily life activities.

One essential principle of yoga is mindfulness. By practicing mindfulness, we become more aware of our thoughts, emotions, and physical sensations. This awareness allows us to make conscious choices throughout the day, promoting overall well-being. Whether we are eating, walking, or simply sitting down to relax, being mindful helps us fully engage in the present moment and appreciate the small joys of life.

Another fundamental principle is breath awareness. The breath is a powerful tool that can be used to reduce stress, increase relaxation, and enhance vitality. By incorporating deep breathing exercises into our daily activities, such as while cooking, gardening, or even watching TV, we can infuse a sense of calm and serenity into our lives.

Yoga also emphasizes the importance of balance and stability. As we age, maintaining balance becomes crucial to prevent falls and injuries. By incorporating simple balance exercises into our daily routines, such as standing on one leg while brushing our teeth or doing heel-to-toe walks while waiting in line, we can strengthen our muscles and improve our overall stability.

Flexibility is another key aspect of yoga that can be integrated into daily life. Simple stretches can be performed while doing household chores, such as reaching up to a high shelf or bending down to pick something up. By incorporating gentle stretches into our daily activities, we can improve our range of motion and prevent muscle stiffness and joint pain.

Finally, the concept of self-care is central to yoga philosophy. Taking time for ourselves, whether it's through meditation, reading a book, or enjoying a warm bath, is essential for our overall well-being. By incorporating self-care activities into our daily routines, we prioritize our own health and happiness.

Incorporating yoga principles into our daily life activities is a powerful way to enhance our overall wellness as seniors. By practicing mindfulness, breath awareness, balance, flexibility, and self-care, we can experience the transformative benefits of yoga throughout our day. Remember, it's never too late to start incorporating these principles into your life and reap the rewards of a holistic and vibrant existence.

Exploring Mindful Movement and Gentle Exercise Option

As we age, it becomes increasingly important to prioritize our physical well-being. Engaging in regular exercise not only helps to maintain a healthy weight and prevent chronic illnesses but also improves flexibility, balance, and overall quality of life. For adults over 60, incorporating mindful movement and gentle exercise options into their routine can be highly beneficial. We will delve into the world of yoga for seniors, exploring various techniques and practices that promote holistic wellness.

Yoga has long been recognized as a powerful tool for physical, mental, and emotional well-being. When tailored specifically for seniors, it offers a gentle yet effective way to maintain and improve strength, flexibility, and balance. Mindful movement is at the core of yoga for seniors, emphasizing slow, controlled motions that allow individuals to connect with their bodies and the present moment.

Chair yoga is an excellent option for those with limited mobility or balance concerns. It adapts traditional yoga poses to be performed while seated or using a chair for support, ensuring safety and accessibility for all. From gentle stretches to breathing exercises, chair yoga offers a full-body workout that can be easily modified to suit individual needs.

For those seeking a more active practice, restorative yoga provides a wonderful opportunity to rejuvenate and relax. This style of yoga involves holding poses for an extended period, allowing the body to release tension and restore energy levels. With the support of props such as bolsters and blankets, seniors can comfortably experience the benefits of deep stretching and gentle movement.

In addition to yoga, other gentle exercise options like Tai Chi and Qigong can enhance overall well-being. These ancient Chinese practices combine slow, fluid movements with focused breathing and meditation, promoting balance, coordination, and mental clarity. Both Tai Chi and Qigong can be easily adapted for seniors, making them ideal choices for those looking to strengthen their bodies and calm their minds.

By exploring mindful movement and gentle exercise options like yoga, Tai Chi, and Qigong, seniors can unlock a multitude of physical and mental benefits. Whether you are a seasoned yogi or a beginner, these practices provide a holistic approach to wellness, allowing you to age gracefully while maintaining a strong and flexible body. Embrace the power of mindful movement and embark on a journey toward a healthier, more vibrant life.

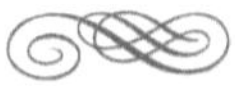

Engaging in Community Yoga Events and Workshops

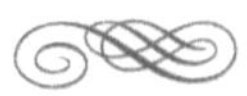

AS WE AGE, IT'S MORE important than ever to stay active and engage in our communities. One fantastic way to achieve this is by participating in community yoga events and workshops specifically designed for seniors. Yoga has been proven to promote holistic wellness, offering a range of physical, mental, and emotional benefits. We will explore the various ways in which engaging in community yoga events and workshops can enhance the lives of adults over 60.

First and foremost, community yoga events provide a wonderful opportunity to meet like-minded individuals who share a common interest in yoga and healthy aging. These events often foster a sense of camaraderie and belonging, creating a supportive community where participants can form new friendships and connections. Engaging in yoga alongside fellow seniors can be a motivating and inspiring experience, as you witness others embracing their own wellness journeys.

Attending workshops specifically tailored for seniors can also deepen your yoga practice and understanding. These workshops are led by experienced instructors who specialize in yoga for seniors, ensuring that the exercises and postures are safe and suitable for your age group. By participating in these workshops, you can learn modifications and adaptions that cater to your unique needs, allowing you to fully enjoy the benefits of yoga without any discomfort or risk of injury.

Chapter Thirteen:

Embracing Holistic Wellness through Yoga

Recap of Key Concepts and Takeaways

As we near the end of our journey through "The Silver Yogi: Holistic Wellness through Yoga for Seniors," it's important to take a moment to reflect on the key concepts and takeaways we have explored so far. We summarize the essential knowledge and insights gained throughout the book, offering a comprehensive recap for our audience of adults over 60 who are interested in practicing yoga for seniors.

First and foremost, we have to emphasize the importance of holistic wellness. Yoga is not just about physical exercise; it encompasses the integration of mind, body, and spirit. By engaging in yoga practice, seniors can experience a wide range of benefits, including improved flexibility, strength, balance, and mental clarity.

One fundamental concept we have explored is the idea that yoga is a practice for everybody. Regardless of age, ability, or limitations, yoga can be adapted to suit individual needs. Modifications and props can be used to ensure each pose is accessible and safe, enabling seniors to reap the rewards of yoga while respecting their unique physical conditions.

Throughout the book, we have delved into various yoga poses and sequences specifically tailored for seniors. From gentle stretches to more challenging postures, each pose has been carefully selected to target common areas of concern for this age group, such as joint mobility, back pain, and overall flexibility. By practicing these poses regularly, seniors can experience increased vitality and a greater sense of well-being.

Furthermore, we have explored the importance of breathwork and meditation in yoga practice. Breathing exercises, such as deep belly breathing and alternative nostril breathing, can help seniors manage stress, improve lung capacity, and enhance overall relaxation. Meditation techniques, such as mindfulness and loving-kindness meditation, can cultivate a sense of inner peace and contentment, allowing seniors to navigate life's challenges with grace and equanimity.

Lastly, we have highlighted the significance of incorporating yoga philosophy into our daily lives. The principles of non-violence, truthfulness, contentment, self-discipline, and self-study can guide us toward living a fulfilling and purposeful life, even in our golden years.

In conclusion, "The Silver Yogi: Holistic Wellness through Yoga for Seniors" has introduced us to the transformative power of yoga for adults over 60. By embracing the key concepts explored throughout this book and incorporating them into our daily lives, we can unlock the potential for enhanced physical health, mental well-being, and spiritual growth. Let us embark on this journey together, embracing the wisdom of yoga and celebrating our silver years with grace and vitality.

Encouragement for Continued Yoga Practice and Growth

Congratulations on embarking on your yoga journey! As adults over 60, you have taken a significant step toward enhancing your overall well-being through the practice of yoga. We will explore some essential elements that will encourage you to continue your yoga practice and foster growth in your journey as a silver yogi.

First and foremost, it is crucial to acknowledge the progress you have already made. Every time you step on your yoga mat, you are investing in your physical, mental, and emotional health. Take a moment to appreciate how far you have come and the positive impact yoga has had on your life. This recognition will serve as a great motivation to keep going.

One of the key aspects of continued yoga practice is setting realistic goals. Remember that yoga is a personal journey, and there is no need to compare yourself to others. Focus on your own progress and set attainable goals that align with your abilities and aspirations. Whether it's mastering a challenging pose or improving flexibility, breaking down your goals into smaller milestones will make them more achievable and enjoyable.

As you progress in your yoga practice, it is essential to embrace the concept of self-compassion. Be gentle with yourself and listen to your body. Honor its limitations and give yourself permission to modify poses or take breaks when needed. Remember, yoga is about finding balance, both physically and mentally. By practicing self-compassion, you are nurturing a positive and sustainable relationship with your body.

To foster growth in your yoga practice, consider expanding your horizons. Explore different styles of yoga and discover what resonates with you the most. Engage in workshops or join a yoga community specifically tailored for seniors. Surrounded yourself with like-minded individuals will not only provide a support system but also offer opportunities for growth and learning.

Lately, remember that yoga is not just a physical practice; it is a holistic approach to wellness. Embrace the mindfulness and spiritual aspects of yoga by incorporating breathing exercises and meditation into your routine. These practices will deepen your connection with yourself and help find inner peace and balance.

In conclusion, as a silver yogi, your journey is a continuous process of growth and self-discovery. By acknowledging your progress, setting realistic goals, practicing self-compassion, exploring new avenues, and embracing the holistic aspects of yoga, you will find not only encouragement. But also immense joy in your continued yoga practice.

Inspiring Seniors to Embrace a Vibrant and Fulfilling Life

As we age, it is easy to fall into the trap of thinking that our best years are behind us. However, nothing could be further from the truth. The journey into our golden years can be a time of incredible growth, joy, and fulfillment. We explore how yoga can help seniors embrace a vibrant and fulfilling life.

Yoga is a practice that transcends age, and its benefits are particularly profound for seniors. It is a holistic approach to wellness that nourishes the mind, body, and spirit. Through gentle movements, breathing exercises, and meditation, yoga offers a path to improved physical health, mental clarity, and emotional well-being.

We delve into the power of yoga to inspire seniors to live their lives to the fullest. We address the unique challenges faced by older adults and provide practical strategies to overcome them. Whether you are new to yoga or have been practicing for years, embrace the transformative potential of this ancient practice.

We start by exploring the physical benefits of yoga for seniors. Regular yoga practice can help improve flexibility, strength, and balance, reducing the risk of falls and injuries. We provide a series of gentle yoga poses specifically tailored for older bodies, ensuring safety and comfort while maximizing the benefits.

Beyond the physical, we delve into the mental and emotional benefits of yoga. As we age, it is common to experience feelings of isolation, loss, and uncertainty. Yoga offers a sanctuary where we can cultivate inner peace, resilience, and a sense of purpose. We discuss mindfulness techniques that can help seniors navigate life's challenges with grace and equanimity.

Additionally, we highlight the importance of community and connection in the lives of seniors. Engaging in yoga classes specifically designed for seniors creates a supportive environment where individuals can build new friendships and share experiences. We emphasize the power of social interaction and encourage seniors to actively seek our opportunities for connection. Remember, age is just a number, and a vibrant and fulfilling life is within reach. By embracing yoga and its holistic approach to wellness, seniors can tap into their inner strength, find renewed purpose, and create a life that is rich with joy and fulfillment.

Don't miss out!

Visit the website below and you can sign up to receive emails whenever Linda Standridge publishes a new book. There's no charge and no obligation.

https://books2read.com/r/B-A-IMCBB-PDKRC

BOOKS 2 READ

Connecting independent readers to independent writers.

About the Author

Linda Standridge is a small-town southern gal. She spends her days fantasizing about sexy aliens or simply writing about sexy aliens. When she isn't doing that she is spending time with her grandchildren and her children. She enjoys gardening and crocheting too. She promises she hasn't lost it entirely. She just loves talking about herself in the third person. She'd love to hear from ya'll.

Give her a shout-out at lindastandridgeauthor@gmail.com